7-Day

Weight Loss

Revolution

Your Fast-Track to a Healthier You

James J. Maas

Copyright © 2023

by James J. Maas

All rights reserved.

Table of Content

Introduction

Welcome to the 7-Day Weight Loss Revolution!

Have you ever found yourself standing in front of the mirror, wishing you could transform your body and your life in just a matter of days? Perhaps you've tried numerous diets, exercise plans, and weight loss schemes, only to feel frustrated by the lack of sustainable results. You're not alone. In a world filled with quick fixes and overnight transformations, it's easy to become disillusioned by the promises of rapid weight loss.

But what if I told you that you could embark on a transformative journey, one that lasts just seven days, and emerge on the other side with not only a slimmer waistline but also renewed energy, enhanced confidence, and a roadmap to lasting health? This is not a fantasy; it's a reality that we're about to embark upon together.

The 7-Day Weight Loss Revolution: Your Fast-Track to a Healthier You is not just another crash diet book that leaves you hungry, tired, and defeated. Instead, it's a holistic guide designed to help you make meaningful and lasting changes to your lifestyle. This journey is not about deprivation or suffering. It's about empowerment, education, and sustainable transformation.

The concept of a "revolution" may conjure images of upheaval and drastic change, and that's precisely what we aim to achieve—but in a healthy, controlled, and supportive way. In just seven days, you'll embark on a journey that will challenge your habits, inspire your choices, and lay the foundation for a healthier, happier you.

Why This Book Is Your Fast-Track to a Healthier You

With the plethora of weight loss advice available today, you might wonder why this book is different. The answer lies in our commitment to combining the latest scientific knowledge with practical, real-world strategies. We've distilled the most effective principles of nutrition, exercise, and behavior change into a seven-day program that's both manageable and transformative.

Our goal isn't just to help you shed pounds temporarily; it's to empower you with the knowledge and tools needed to maintain a healthy weight and lifestyle long after these seven days are over. We want you to experience the joy of discovering a healthier, happier, and more energetic you—a version of yourself that you can be proud of and sustain for years to come.

The Importance of Sustainable Weight Loss

Before we dive into the specifics of this program, it's essential to understand the significance of sustainable weight loss. We're not interested in promoting extreme diets or quick fixes that might lead to temporary results but ultimately harm your health and well-being. Instead, we emphasize the importance of creating lasting change through realistic and science-backed methods.

Over the next seven days, you'll learn how to nourish your body with the right foods, move it effectively through exercise, and develop a mindset that supports your goals. This isn't just about losing weight; it's about gaining health, confidence, and a brighter outlook on life.

So, are you ready to embark on this exciting journey? If you're tired of fad diets, unsustainable exercise regimens, and empty promises, then fasten your seatbelt because we're about to take a seven-day ride that will transform the way you think about weight loss and health.

Get ready to embark on the 7-Day Weight Loss Revolution and discover the healthier you that's been waiting to emerge. It's time to rewrite your story, and it begins right here, right now.

Let's revolutionize your life, one day at a time.

Chapter 1

Setting the Stage

Imagine yourself standing at the starting line of a race. You're here because you've decided it's time for a change—a change that will lead you to a healthier, happier, and more confident you. This race isn't measured in miles or kilometers; it's a journey that spans just seven days. Welcome to the 7-Day Weight Loss Revolution, where we'll set the stage for your transformation.

Understanding Your Current Health and Lifestyle

Before we dive headfirst into the action, it's essential to take a moment to understand where you currently stand. Just as a navigator needs to know their starting point to chart a course to their destination, you need to assess your current health and lifestyle to embark on a successful weight loss journey.

Self-Assessment: Where Are You Now?

Take a moment to reflect on your current habits and health:

- What is your current weight, and how do you feel about it?
- How is your energy level throughout the day?
- Are you satisfied with your current eating habits?
- Do you engage in regular physical activity?
- How do you handle stress, and how well do you sleep?

By honestly assessing your starting point, you gain valuable insight into the factors that have led you to this moment. Remember, this isn't about judgment; it's about understanding.

Goal Setting: What Do You Want to Achieve in 7 Days?

Now that you have a clear picture of where you're starting from, it's time to set your sights on your destination. In just seven days, what do you hope to achieve? Your goals will serve as your guiding star throughout this journey, helping you stay focused and motivated.

S.M.A.R.T. Goals for Success

- Specific: Clearly define what you want to accomplish.
- Measurable: Establish concrete criteria to track your progress.

- Achievable: Set realistic and attainable goals.
- Relevant: Ensure your goals align with your overall health and well-being.
- Time-bound: Set a specific timeframe for achieving your goals.

Perhaps your goals include losing a certain number of pounds, increasing your daily step count, or making healthier food choices. Whatever they may be, write them down and keep them in a place where you can revisit them daily.

Creating a Positive Mindset for Success

As you embark on this 7-day journey, your mindset will be your most powerful asset. A positive mindset can propel you forward when faced with challenges and temptations. It's the unwavering belief that you have the capability to achieve your goals, no matter the obstacles.

The Power of Positivity

- Cultivate self-compassion: Be kind to yourself, and don't let setbacks define your journey.
- Visualization: Imagine your success and how it will feel.

- Affirmations: Use positive affirmations to reinforce your belief in yourself.

Your mindset isn't just about thinking positively; it's about fostering self-belief and resilience. Remember, you have the power to make lasting changes in your life, and it all starts with the belief that you can.

Chapter 2

The Science of Weight Loss

In our quest for lasting weight loss and a healthier life, knowledge is power. Understanding the science behind weight loss arms us with the tools and insights necessary to make informed decisions, set realistic expectations, and ultimately achieve our goals. So, let's dive into the science of weight loss, demystify the process, and lay the groundwork for your transformative journey.

Demystifying Calories and Metabolism

The Caloric Equation At the core of weight loss lies the simple principle of calories in versus calories out. In other words, you lose weight when you burn more calories than you consume. This forms the foundation of our journey. But remember, it's not just about cutting calories; it's about making wise choices.

Metabolism: Your Body's Engine Your metabolism is the engine that burns calories to fuel your body's functions. It consists of your Basal Metabolic Rate

(BMR) and the calories burned through physical activity and digestion. Understanding your metabolism helps you tailor your approach to weight loss to your unique needs.

The Role of Nutrition and Exercise

Nutrition: Fueling Your Body Right The food you eat isn't just about satisfying hunger; it's about providing essential nutrients that support your health and well-being. We'll explore the importance of balanced nutrition and delve into the macronutrients—carbohydrates, proteins, and fats—and how they contribute to your weight loss goals.

Exercise: Boosting Your Caloric Burn Physical activity is a key component of your weight loss journey. It not only burns calories but also strengthens your body and boosts your metabolism. We'll discuss different types of exercise, from cardio to strength training, and how to incorporate them into your daily routine.

How Stress and Sleep Affect Weight

Stress: The Silent Saboteur Stress can derail your weight loss efforts by triggering emotional eating and disrupting your hormones. We'll explore stress management techniques that help you stay on track.

The Importance of Sleep Sleep is a powerful ally in weight loss. Poor sleep can lead to weight gain by affecting hunger hormones and increasing cravings. Discover strategies for improving your sleep quality and duration.

As we wrap up this chapter, remember that knowledge is the first step toward lasting change. You now have a foundational understanding of the science behind weight loss, from calories and metabolism to the roles of nutrition, exercise, stress, and sleep.

Chapter 3

Preparing for Your 7-Day Journey

As you stand on the precipice of your 7-Day Weight Loss Revolution, the key to your success lies in preparation. Just as a chef organizes their ingredients before creating a masterpiece, we must prepare our environment and mindset for the transformative week ahead. In this chapter, we'll explore the essential steps to ensure you're ready for your journey.

Cleaning Out Your Pantry and Fridge

Out with the Old Begin your preparation by conducting a pantry and fridge overhaul. Remove tempting, unhealthy items that could derail your progress. Out of sight, out of mind. Instead, stock your kitchen with nutritious options that align with your goals.

Label Reading 101 Understanding food labels empowers you to make informed choices. Learn to decipher the nutrition facts panel and ingredient list to select healthier options.

Grocery Shopping for Success

The Art of Meal Planning Before hitting the grocery store, plan your meals for the week. A well-thought-out meal plan ensures you have the right ingredients on hand, reducing the temptation to order takeout or opt for unhealthy choices.

Shopping with Purpose Stick to your shopping list to avoid impulsive purchases. Load up on fresh produce, lean proteins, whole grains, and other staples that feature prominently in your meal plan.

Smart Snacking Choose healthy snacks to keep on hand. Pre-cut veggies, nuts, and yogurt are excellent options to satisfy between-meal cravings.

Meal Planning and Preparation Tips

Batch Cooking Spend a day batch-cooking meals for the week. This not only saves time but also ensures you have nutritious options readily available when you're pressed for time.

Portion Control Use portion control tools like measuring cups and a food scale to avoid overeating. Being mindful of portion sizes is crucial for success.

Stay Hydrated Don't forget about hydration. Drinking enough water is essential for overall health and can help curb appetite.

In this chapter, you've laid the groundwork for your 7-Day Weight Loss Revolution by preparing your kitchen and pantry for success. You've learned to read labels, make strategic grocery choices, and plan and prepare your meals with intention.

Preparation is the secret ingredient that will make your journey smoother and more enjoyable. By setting up your environment for success, you've taken a significant step toward achieving your goals. Now, with your kitchen in order and your mindset focused, you're ready to kick off Day 1 of your transformative week. Get ready to put your preparation into action and take the first step toward a healthier you. The 7-Day Weight Loss Revolution is about to begin.

Chapter 4

The 7-Day Meal Plan

Welcome to the heart of your 7-Day Weight Loss Revolution—the meal plan that will guide you through seven days of nourishing your body, boosting your metabolism, and propelling you toward your goals. Each day is meticulously designed to ensure you get the nutrients you need while enjoying delicious, satisfying meals.

Day 1: Kickstart Your Journey

Breakfast: Energizing Smoothie

- Packed with fiber, protein, and antioxidants to jumpstart your metabolism.

Lunch: Grilled Chicken Salad

- A balanced meal with lean protein, veggies, and a light dressing.

Dinner: Baked Salmon with Quinoa and Steamed Broccoli

- Omega-3-rich salmon, whole grains, and fiber-packed broccoli.

Snack: Greek Yogurt with Berries

- A protein-rich snack to keep your energy levels stable.

Day 2: Fueling Your Body Right

Breakfast: Overnight Oats with Almond Butter and Banana

- A hearty breakfast that provides long-lasting energy.

Lunch: Turkey and Avocado Wrap

- Lean protein and healthy fats for a satisfying midday meal.

Dinner: Stir-Fried Tofu with Vegetables and Brown Rice

- Plant-based protein and fiber-rich grains and veggies.

Snack: Sliced Cucumbers with Hummus

- A crunchy, nutrient-packed snack.

Day 3: Boosting Your Metabolism

Breakfast: Scrambled Eggs with Spinach and Tomatoes

- Protein and greens to fire up your metabolism.

Lunch: Quinoa Salad with Chickpeas and Veggies

- A plant-based meal rich in protein and fiber.

Dinner: Grilled Shrimp with Asparagus and Quinoa

- Lean protein, fiber, and vitamins.

Snack: Mixed Nuts

- Healthy fats and protein to keep you satisfied.

Day 4: Managing Cravings and Hunger

Breakfast: Whole Grain Pancakes with Berries and Greek Yogurt

- Fiber and protein to curb morning cravings.

Lunch: Lentil Soup with a Side Salad

- A fiber and protein combo to keep you full.

Dinner: Baked Chicken Breast with Sweet Potato and Green Beans

- Lean protein, complex carbs, and fiber.

Snack: Apple Slices with Peanut Butter

- A satisfying and sweet treat.

Day 5: Incorporating Exercise

Breakfast: Protein-Packed Breakfast Burrito

- Fuel for your workout with eggs, veggies, and lean protein.

Lunch: Tuna Salad Lettuce Wraps

- A light, protein-rich lunch to support your active day.

Dinner: Beef and Vegetable Stir-Fry with Brown Rice

- Protein, fiber, and essential nutrients.

Snack: Cottage Cheese with Pineapple

- A protein-packed, post-workout snack.

Day 6: Staying Motivated

Breakfast: Berry and Spinach Smoothie Bowl

- Antioxidants and protein to keep you motivated.

Lunch: Turkey and Veggie Stir-Fry

- Lean protein and colorful veggies for energy.

Dinner: Baked Cod with Quinoa and Steamed Asparagus

- Lean protein, fiber, and essential nutrients.

Snack: Carrot Sticks with Hummus

- A crunchy, satisfying snack.

Day 7: Celebrating Your Success

Breakfast: Veggie Omelette with Whole Wheat Toast

- A balanced breakfast to kickstart your day.

Lunch: Spinach and Feta Stuffed Chicken Breast with a Side Salad

- Lean protein and greens for a special occasion.

Dinner: Grilled Steak with Roasted Vegetables and Quinoa

- Protein, fiber, and a satisfying indulgence.

Snack: Dark Chocolate Square

- A small treat to celebrate your success.

Important Note

Remember to drink plenty of water throughout the day to stay hydrated and support your metabolism. Additionally, portion control is key. Be mindful of portion sizes to avoid overeating.

This 7-Day Meal Plan is your roadmap to success during your weight loss journey. It's designed to provide you with the nutrients you need while keeping you satisfied and energized. Each meal and snack has a purpose—to fuel your body, curb cravings, and support your goals.

As you dive into these meals over the coming week, keep in mind the larger picture. This isn't just about what you eat; it's about forming healthier eating habits that can extend far beyond these seven days. Embrace this meal plan as a tool to nourish your body and revitalize your health.

With your meal plan in hand, you're now ready to embark on the first day of your 7-Day Weight Loss Revolution. Your journey to a healthier you begins now.

Chapter 5

Exercise for Weight Loss

In this chapter, we're diving headfirst into the world of exercise—a crucial component of your 7-Day Weight Loss Revolution. While nutrition plays a significant role in weight management, exercise is the dynamic force that accelerates your progress, tones your body, and boosts your metabolism. Let's explore how to incorporate effective exercise into your daily routine.

The Importance of Physical Activity

Beyond the Scale Exercise isn't just about the number on the scale. It's about how you feel, your energy levels, and your overall well-being. Regular physical activity has a profound impact on your health, extending far beyond weight loss.

Weight Loss Benefits

- Burns calories: Exercise increases your energy expenditure, aiding in weight loss.
- Preserves muscle mass: Exercise helps maintain lean muscle, which is essential for a higher metabolism.

- Improves mood: Physical activity releases endorphins, reducing stress and enhancing your mood.
- Enhances overall health: Exercise reduces the risk of chronic diseases like heart disease and diabetes.

The 7-Day Exercise Plan for All Fitness Levels

Day 1: Walk It Out

- Start with a brisk 30-minute walk. It's gentle yet effective for beginners.

Day 2: Strength Training

- Basic bodyweight exercises like squats, push-ups, and planks for 20 minutes.

Day 3: Cardio Blast

- A 20-minute interval workout, alternating between high-intensity and low-intensity bursts.

Day 4: Rest and Recovery

- Your body needs time to recover. Rest or do gentle stretching.

Day 5: Total Body Workout

- A mix of bodyweight exercises and light dumbbell work for 30 minutes.

Day 6: Cardio Fun

- Engage in an activity you enjoy, whether it's dancing, cycling, or swimming for 30 minutes.

Day 7: Yoga and Relaxation

- 20 minutes of yoga to improve flexibility and reduce stress.

Incorporating Movement into Your Daily Life

Active Living

- Find opportunities to move throughout the day, such as taking the stairs, stretching breaks, and short walks.

Set Realistic Goals

- Gradually increase the intensity and duration of your workouts as you build strength and stamina.

Stay Consistent

- Consistency is key to reaping the benefits of exercise. Make it a daily habit.

Exercise is the catalyst that propels your weight loss journey forward, and it offers numerous other health benefits beyond shedding pounds. By incorporating physical activity into your daily life, you're not only sculpting your body but also boosting your mood and improving your overall well-being.

As you follow the 7-Day Exercise Plan, remember that fitness is a journey, not a destination. The goal isn't to become an Olympic athlete in a week; it's to establish a foundation of regular physical activity that you can build upon in the weeks and months ahead.

Whether you're a seasoned athlete or new to exercise, this chapter has something to offer. The most important thing is to move your body regularly and make exercise an integral part of your lifestyle.

With exercise as your ally, you're now fully equipped to conquer Day 1 of your 7-Day Weight Loss Revolution. Get ready to feel the burn, build strength, and invigorate your journey to a healthier you. Your transformative week continues, fueled by the power of movement.

Chapter 6

Overcoming Challenges

In the midst of any journey, challenges are bound to arise. Your 7-Day Weight Loss Revolution is no exception. However, it's how you face and overcome these challenges that truly defines your success. In this chapter, we'll explore common obstacles and provide strategies to navigate them effectively.

Dealing with Plateaus

The Plateau Dilemma It's not uncommon to hit a plateau where your weight loss stalls despite your efforts. Plateaus can be frustrating, but they're a natural part of the process.

Plateau-Busting Strategies

- Reevaluate your calorie intake and adjust if necessary.
- Vary your workouts to prevent adaptation.
- Focus on non-scale victories, such as improved energy and fitness levels.

Managing Emotional Eating

The Emotional Eating Connection

Emotional eating is a common coping mechanism. Stress, boredom, and even happiness can trigger overeating or unhealthy food choices.

Strategies to Combat Emotional Eating

- Identify emotional triggers and develop alternative coping mechanisms like journaling or talking to a friend.
- Practice mindful eating to stay present and aware of your food choices.

- Stock your kitchen with healthy comfort foods for when cravings strike.

Staying Consistent Beyond the 7 Days

The Transition to Long-Term Success Completing the 7-Day Weight Loss Revolution is a significant achievement, but the real challenge lies in maintaining your progress.

Strategies for Long-Term Success

- Gradually reintroduce a wider variety of foods into your diet while maintaining portion control.

- Continue with regular exercise, adjusting your routine to keep it interesting.
- Set new goals to keep your motivation high.

Challenges are not roadblocks; they are opportunities for growth. In your 7-Day Weight Loss Revolution, you will face hurdles, but with the right strategies, you can overcome them. Remember that perfection is not the goal—progress is.

By acknowledging plateaus, managing emotional eating, and focusing on long-term success, you're equipping yourself with the tools to navigate the inevitable bumps in the road. Weight loss is a journey, not a destination, and your resilience in the face of challenges is what will truly lead you to lasting success.

With these strategies in your arsenal, you're ready to face whatever challenges come your way on your 7-Day Weight Loss Revolution. As you continue your transformative week, remember that every setback is a setup for a comeback. You've got this!

Chapter 7

Tracking Your Progress

Tracking your progress is like navigating with a map—it keeps you on course and helps you stay motivated on your 7-Day Weight Loss Revolution. In this chapter, we'll explore the importance of monitoring your journey, different methods of tracking, and celebrating milestones along the way.

The Power of Journaling

Why Journaling Matters Keeping a journal provides insight into your habits, triggers, and progress. It's your personal record of your weight loss journey.

What to Include in Your Journal

- Daily food intake: Document everything you eat and drink.
- Exercise routines: Note the type, duration, and intensity of your workouts.
- Emotions and triggers: Record how you feel and what may be influencing your choices.

- Measurements and milestones: Track your weight, body measurements, and other achievements.

Using Technology for Monitoring

Mobile Apps and Devices In today's digital age, there are numerous apps and devices designed to help you track your weight loss journey with precision.

Benefits of Technology

- Real-time tracking: Many apps sync with wearables for immediate data.
- Data analysis: Charts and graphs provide visual feedback on your progress.
- Accountability: Some apps offer community support and challenges.

Celebrating Milestones

Why Milestones Matter Milestones are not just for major achievements; they help you acknowledge your progress, no matter how small.

Types of Milestones

- Scale victories: Celebrate weight loss milestones.
- Non-scale victories: Recognize improvements in energy, fitness, and overall health.
- Behavioral milestones: Reward yourself for consistently making healthy choices.

Staying Motivated

Visual Reminders Create visual reminders of your progress to stay motivated. This can be a "before and after" photo, a vision board, or a list of your goals.

Rewards and Treats Consider rewards for reaching milestones, but make them non-food-related. Treat yourself to a massage, a new book, or a spa day.

Accountability Partners Share your journey with a friend or family member who can hold you accountable and celebrate your successes with you.

Tracking your progress is an essential aspect of your 7-Day Weight Loss Revolution. It provides clarity, motivation, and a sense of achievement as you work toward your goals. Whether you prefer journaling, technology, or a combination of both, the act of monitoring your journey keeps you engaged and accountable.

As you embark on your transformative week, remember that every step you take, every healthy choice you make, is a move in the right direction. By tracking your progress and celebrating milestones along the way, you're not only achieving your weight loss goals but also building a foundation for a healthier, happier future.

Stay committed, stay accountable, and keep moving forward. Your journey is a testament to your dedication and resilience. The best is yet to come.

Chapter 8

Maintaining Your Weight Loss

Congratulations on completing your 7-Day Weight Loss Revolution! As you stand on the precipice of your journey's conclusion, it's essential to recognize that maintaining your weight loss is just as crucial as achieving it. In this chapter, we'll explore the strategies and habits that will help you sustain your newfound health and well-being.

Transitioning to a Sustainable Lifestyle

The Post-Revolution Phase Your 7-Day Weight Loss Revolution may be over, but your journey is far from finished. The next steps are about transitioning from a short-term plan to a sustainable lifestyle.

Gradual Reintroduction of Foods Start incorporating a wider variety of foods into your diet while maintaining portion control. This allows you to enjoy a balanced and enjoyable way of eating.

Finding Your Maintenance Caloric Intake Determine the number of calories you need to maintain your current weight. This can be done through trial and error while monitoring your weight and adjusting your caloric intake accordingly.

Long-Term Strategies for Success

Mindful Eating Continue practicing mindful eating, which involves paying attention to your hunger cues, savoring your food, and eating without distractions. This helps prevent overeating.

Regular Exercise Maintain your exercise routine, adjusting it to your goals. Whether it's maintaining your current weight or pursuing new fitness goals, exercise remains a cornerstone of your healthy lifestyle.

Stress Management and Sleep Keep managing stress through relaxation techniques, hobbies, and activities you enjoy. Prioritize sleep to ensure you're well-rested and able to make healthy choices.

Staying Inspired and Motivated

Setting New Goals Once you've achieved your initial weight loss goals, it's time to set new ones. These can be fitness-related, such as running a 5k, or health-oriented, like reducing your risk of chronic diseases.

Community and Support Stay connected with others who share your goals. Join fitness classes, engage in online communities, or find a workout buddy. Support and accountability can be powerful motivators.

Rewarding Yourself Celebrate your successes along the way. Whether it's reaching a maintenance milestone or achieving a new fitness goal, acknowledge your accomplishments with non-food rewards.

Maintaining your weight loss is the true measure of success. It's about embracing a new way of life that prioritizes health, well-being, and self-care. While the 7-Day Weight Loss Revolution served as a catalyst for change, the habits and strategies you've cultivated during this journey will serve you for years to come.

As you move forward, remember that setbacks are a natural part of any journey, but they don't define your destination.

Your commitment to your health and well-being remains unwavering. By transitioning to a sustainable lifestyle, employing long-term strategies, and staying motivated, you're not only maintaining your weight loss but also setting the stage for a lifetime of health and happiness.

Your 7-Day Weight Loss Revolution was just the beginning of your transformation. Embrace this new chapter with confidence, knowing that you have the tools and knowledge to lead a healthier, happier life. Your journey is now a lifelong adventure, and the possibilities are endless.

Chapter 9

Your Health and Wellness Beyond Weight Loss

As you wrap up your 7-Day Weight Loss Revolution, it's time to shift the spotlight from just the number on the scale to your overall health and well-being. In this chapter, we'll explore how your journey goes far beyond weight loss, encompassing holistic health and lasting wellness.

The Bigger Picture

Beyond the Scale Your journey isn't solely about pounds lost. It's about feeling better, living longer, and enjoying a higher quality of life.

Holistic Health Consider the multiple dimensions of wellness: physical, mental, emotional, and social. Your goal is to thrive in each area.

Physical Health

Increased Energy With your healthier habits, you'll experience improved energy levels. Use this vitality to engage in activities you love.

Reduced Risk of Chronic Diseases Weight loss and a healthier lifestyle can decrease your risk of chronic diseases such as heart disease, diabetes, and hypertension.

Enhanced Fitness Your increased activity level will contribute to improved cardiovascular fitness, strength, and flexibility.

Mental and Emotional Well-Being

Improved Mood Exercise releases endorphins, the body's natural mood boosters. You'll likely notice increased positivity and reduced stress.

Enhanced Confidence Achieving your weight loss goals enhances self-esteem and self-confidence, leading to a more fulfilling life.

Resilience The strategies you've learned during your journey, such as stress management and mindfulness, will serve you well in managing life's challenges.

Social Connections

Community Joining fitness classes, online groups, or workout buddies fosters a sense of belonging and support.

Shared Goals Connecting with others who prioritize health and well-being creates a network of shared goals and motivation.

Setting New Wellness Goals

Lifelong Learning Health and wellness are ongoing journeys. Continue to educate yourself about nutrition, exercise, and stress management.

New Adventures Set new wellness goals, such as trying a new sport, participating in a charity run, or exploring different types of exercise.

Giving Back Share your knowledge and journey with others. Consider becoming a mentor or supporting a friend in their wellness endeavors.

Your 7-Day Weight Loss Revolution is a springboard to a lifetime of health and well-being. As you move forward, remember that your journey is not a destination but an ongoing adventure. It's about more than just numbers on a scale; it's about experiencing life to the fullest, with vitality and vigor.

With the tools, strategies, and insights gained during this transformative week, you're equipped to embrace a holistic approach to health. By prioritizing your physical, mental, emotional, and social well-being, you're creating a life that's rich in fulfillment, joy, and longevity.

As you embark on this lifelong journey, savor every moment, celebrate your victories, and stay committed to your health and wellness. The 7-Day Weight Loss Revolution was just the beginning—your life of vibrant well-being awaits, and the possibilities are boundless.

Conclusion

Your Journey, Your Revolution

As you close the final chapter of "7-Day Weight Loss Revolution: Your Fast-Track to a Healthier You," take a moment to reflect on the incredible journey you've embarked upon. You've traveled from the starting line, armed with determination and curiosity, to a place of empowerment, knowledge, and transformation. But this journey is far from over; in fact, it's only just beginning.

A Revolution of Self-Discovery

Your journey wasn't just about shedding pounds; it was a voyage of self-discovery. You learned that lasting change starts from within, fueled by your belief in yourself and your unwavering commitment to health and well-being. You discovered that the power of transformation lies not only in the food you eat and the exercise you do but also in the way you think and the choices you make.

Beyond the Scale

Your 7-Day Weight Loss Revolution wasn't merely about the numbers on a scale. It was a holistic experience that transcended weight loss, encompassing every facet of your health and wellness. You realized that vitality, energy, and a zest for life are as crucial as any numerical measurement. Your journey was a testament to the interconnectedness of physical, mental, emotional, and social well-being.

The Power of Habits

Throughout your journey, you've cultivated healthy habits that have become an integral part of your life. You've learned the art of meal planning, the science of exercise, and the importance of tracking your progress. These habits are your tools for lifelong health and wellness, guiding you through the twists and turns of your ongoing adventure.

The End Is Just the Beginning

As you conclude this chapter and close the book, remember that the end of one chapter marks the beginning of the next. Your 7-Day Weight Loss Revolution was not a finite journey but a stepping stone to a lifetime of health and happiness. Your future is filled with opportunities to set new goals, explore new horizons, and inspire others on their paths to wellness.

Embrace Your Revolution

Your transformation is an ongoing revolution—an evolution of self-improvement and self-care. It's about nourishing your body with wholesome foods, nurturing your mind with positive thoughts, and cherishing your spirit with gratitude and purpose. It's about being kind to yourself and celebrating every step forward, no matter how small.

Your Journey Continues

As you embark on the next phase of your journey, carry with you the knowledge that you are the author of your story, the captain of your ship, and the architect of your destiny. Your 7-Day Weight Loss Revolution was just the beginning—a foundation upon which to build a life filled with health, joy, and vitality.

Your journey continues, your revolution persists, and the possibilities are limitless. Embrace each day as a chance to live your best life, and remember that your potential for greatness knows no bounds.

Thank you for allowing this book to be a part of your journey. May your path be paved with wellness, and may your revolution be a beacon of inspiration for others. Your transformation is a testament to the incredible power that resides within you. Keep moving forward, and embrace the vibrant, healthy, and fulfilling life that awaits you.